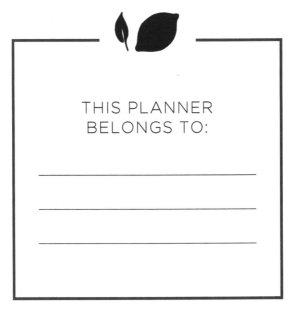

THIS PLANNER
BELONGS TO:

_____

_____

_____

BON APPÉTIT!

MONDAY

....

TUESDAY

....

WEDNESDAY

....

THURSDAY

....

FRIDAY

....

SATURDAY

....

SUNDAY

....

MEAL PLAN FOR THE WEEK OF:

BREAKFAST IDEAS

LUNCH IDEAS

SHOPPING LIST

DELISH!

MONDAY ....

TUESDAY ....

WEDNESDAY ....

THURSDAY ....

FRIDAY ....

SATURDAY ....

SUNDAY ....

MEAL PLAN FOR THE WEEK OF:

BREAKFAST IDEAS

_____
_____
_____
_____
_____
_____
_____

LUNCH IDEAS

_____
_____
_____
_____
_____
_____
_____

SHOPPING LIST

NOM NOM NOM!

MONDAY ....

TUESDAY ....

WEDNESDAY ....

THURSDAY ....

FRIDAY ....

SATURDAY ....

SUNDAY ....

MEAL PLAN FOR THE WEEK OF:

BREAKFAST IDEAS

LUNCH IDEAS

SHOPPING LIST

SO TASTY! ▬▬▬

MONDAY ....

_____
_____
_____

TUESDAY ....

_____
_____
_____

WEDNESDAY ....

_____
_____
_____

THURSDAY ....

_____
_____
_____

FRIDAY ....

_____
_____
_____

SATURDAY ....

_____
_____
_____

SUNDAY ....

_____
_____
_____

MEAL PLAN FOR THE WEEK OF:

BREAKFAST IDEAS

LUNCH IDEAS

SHOPPING LIST

BON APPÉTIT! ■

MONDAY ·

_____

_____

_____

TUESDAY ·

_____

_____

_____

WEDNESDAY ·

_____

_____

_____

THURSDAY ·

_____

_____

_____

FRIDAY ·

_____

_____

_____

SATURDAY ·

_____

_____

_____

SUNDAY ·

_____

_____

_____

MEAL PLAN FOR THE WEEK OF:

BREAKFAST IDEAS

LUNCH IDEAS

SHOPPING LIST

DELISH!

MONDAY . . . .

_____

_____

_____

TUESDAY . . . .

_____

_____

_____

WEDNESDAY . . . .

_____

_____

_____

THURSDAY . . . .

_____

_____

_____

FRIDAY . . . .

_____

_____

_____

SATURDAY . . . .

_____

_____

_____

SUNDAY . . . .

_____

_____

_____

MEAL PLAN FOR THE WEEK OF:

BREAKFAST IDEAS

LUNCH IDEAS

SHOPPING LIST

NOM NOM NOM!

MONDAY ....

_____

_____

_____

TUESDAY ....

_____

_____

_____

WEDNESDAY ....

_____

_____

_____

THURSDAY ....

_____

_____

_____

FRIDAY ....

_____

_____

_____

SATURDAY ....

_____

_____

_____

SUNDAY ....

_____

_____

_____

MEAL PLAN FOR THE WEEK OF:

BREAKFAST IDEAS

_____
_____
_____
_____
_____
_____
_____
_____
_____
_____

LUNCH IDEAS

_____
_____
_____
_____
_____
_____
_____
_____
_____
_____

SHOPPING LIST

_____   _____
_____   _____
_____   _____
_____   _____
_____   _____
_____   _____
_____   _____
_____   _____
_____   _____
_____   _____
_____   _____
_____   _____
_____   _____
_____   _____
_____   _____
_____   _____
_____   _____
_____   _____

SO TASTY!

MONDAY
....

_____
_____
_____

TUESDAY
....

_____
_____
_____

WEDNESDAY
....

_____
_____
_____

THURSDAY
....

_____
_____
_____

FRIDAY
....

_____
_____
_____

SATURDAY
....

_____
_____
_____

SUNDAY
....

_____
_____
_____

MEAL PLAN FOR THE WEEK OF:

BREAKFAST IDEAS

LUNCH IDEAS

SHOPPING LIST

BON APPÉTIT!

MONDAY ....

_____
_____
_____

TUESDAY ....

_____
_____
_____

WEDNESDAY ....

_____
_____
_____

THURSDAY ....

_____
_____
_____

FRIDAY ....

_____
_____
_____

SATURDAY ....

_____
_____
_____

SUNDAY ....

_____
_____
_____

MEAL PLAN FOR THE WEEK OF:

BREAKFAST IDEAS

LUNCH IDEAS

SHOPPING LIST

DELISH!

MONDAY ....

_____

_____

_____

TUESDAY ....

_____

_____

_____

WEDNESDAY ....

_____

_____

_____

THURSDAY ....

_____

_____

_____

FRIDAY ....

_____

_____

_____

SATURDAY ....

_____

_____

_____

SUNDAY ....

_____

_____

_____

MEAL PLAN FOR THE WEEK OF:

BREAKFAST IDEAS

LUNCH IDEAS

SHOPPING LIST

NOM NOM NOM!

MONDAY ....

_____

_____

_____

TUESDAY ....

_____

_____

_____

WEDNESDAY ....

_____

_____

_____

THURSDAY ....

_____

_____

_____

FRIDAY ....

_____

_____

_____

SATURDAY ....

_____

_____

_____

SUNDAY ....

_____

_____

_____

MEAL PLAN FOR THE WEEK OF:

BREAKFAST IDEAS

LUNCH IDEAS

SHOPPING LIST

SO TASTY! ▬▬▬▬▬

MONDAY
....

TUESDAY
....

WEDNESDAY
....

THURSDAY
....

FRIDAY
....

SATURDAY
....

SUNDAY
....

MEAL PLAN FOR THE WEEK OF:

BREAKFAST IDEAS

_____
_____
_____
_____
_____
_____
_____
_____
_____

LUNCH IDEAS

_____
_____
_____
_____
_____
_____
_____
_____
_____

SHOPPING LIST

_____   _____
_____   _____
_____   _____
_____   _____
_____   _____
_____   _____
_____   _____
_____   _____
_____   _____
_____   _____
_____   _____
_____   _____
_____   _____
_____   _____
_____   _____
_____   _____
_____   _____

BON APPÉTIT!

MONDAY ....

_____

_____

_____

TUESDAY ....

_____

_____

_____

WEDNESDAY ....

_____

_____

_____

THURSDAY ....

_____

_____

_____

FRIDAY ....

_____

_____

_____

SATURDAY ....

_____

_____

_____

SUNDAY ....

_____

_____

_____

MEAL PLAN FOR THE WEEK OF:

BREAKFAST IDEAS

LUNCH IDEAS

SHOPPING LIST

DELISH! ▬▬▬▬▬

MONDAY ....
_____
_____
_____

TUESDAY ....
_____
_____
_____

WEDNESDAY ....
_____
_____
_____

THURSDAY ....
_____
_____
_____

FRIDAY ....
_____
_____
_____

SATURDAY ....
_____
_____
_____

SUNDAY ....
_____
_____
_____

MEAL PLAN FOR THE WEEK OF:

BREAKFAST IDEAS

LUNCH IDEAS

SHOPPING LIST

NOM NOM NOM!

MONDAY ....

_____
_____
_____

TUESDAY ....

_____
_____
_____

WEDNESDAY ....

_____
_____
_____

THURSDAY ....

_____
_____
_____

FRIDAY ....

_____
_____
_____

SATURDAY ....

_____
_____
_____

SUNDAY ....

_____
_____
_____

MEAL PLAN FOR THE WEEK OF:

BREAKFAST IDEAS

LUNCH IDEAS

SHOPPING LIST

SO TASTY!

MONDAY
....

_____
_____
_____

TUESDAY
....

_____
_____
_____

WEDNESDAY
....

_____
_____
_____

THURSDAY
....

_____
_____
_____

FRIDAY
....

_____
_____
_____

SATURDAY
....

_____
_____
_____

SUNDAY
....

_____
_____
_____

MEAL PLAN FOR THE WEEK OF:

BREAKFAST IDEAS

LUNCH IDEAS

SHOPPING LIST

BON APPÉTIT!

MONDAY

....

_____

_____

_____

TUESDAY

....

_____

_____

_____

WEDNESDAY

....

_____

_____

_____

THURSDAY

....

_____

_____

_____

FRIDAY

....

_____

_____

_____

SATURDAY

....

_____

_____

_____

SUNDAY

....

_____

_____

_____

MEAL PLAN FOR THE WEEK OF:

BREAKFAST IDEAS

LUNCH IDEAS

SHOPPING LIST

DELISH!

MONDAY ....

_____

_____

_____

TUESDAY ....

_____

_____

_____

WEDNESDAY ....

_____

_____

_____

THURSDAY ....

_____

_____

_____

FRIDAY ....

_____

_____

_____

SATURDAY ....

_____

_____

_____

SUNDAY ....

_____

_____

_____

MEAL PLAN FOR THE WEEK OF:

BREAKFAST IDEAS

LUNCH IDEAS

SHOPPING LIST

NOM NOM NOM!

MONDAY . . . .

TUESDAY . . . .

WEDNESDAY . . . .

THURSDAY . . . .

FRIDAY . . . .

SATURDAY . . . .

SUNDAY . . . .

MEAL PLAN FOR THE WEEK OF:

BREAKFAST IDEAS

LUNCH IDEAS

SHOPPING LIST

SO TASTY!

MONDAY ·

TUESDAY ·

WEDNESDAY ·

THURSDAY ·

FRIDAY ·

SATURDAY ·

SUNDAY ·

MEAL PLAN FOR THE WEEK OF:

BREAKFAST IDEAS

LUNCH IDEAS

SHOPPING LIST

BON APPÉTIT! ■

MONDAY
....

_____
_____
_____

TUESDAY
....

_____
_____
_____

WEDNESDAY
....

_____
_____
_____

THURSDAY
....

_____
_____
_____

FRIDAY
....

_____
_____
_____

SATURDAY
....

_____
_____
_____

SUNDAY
....

_____
_____
_____

MEAL PLAN FOR THE WEEK OF:

BREAKFAST IDEAS

LUNCH IDEAS

SHOPPING LIST

DELISH!

MONDAY
....

_____
_____
_____

TUESDAY
....

_____
_____
_____

WEDNESDAY
....

_____
_____
_____

THURSDAY
....

_____
_____
_____

FRIDAY
....

_____
_____
_____

SATURDAY
....

_____
_____
_____

SUNDAY
....

_____
_____
_____

MEAL PLAN FOR THE WEEK OF:

BREAKFAST IDEAS

LUNCH IDEAS

SHOPPING LIST

NOM NOM NOM!

MONDAY ....

TUESDAY ....

WEDNESDAY ....

THURSDAY ....

FRIDAY ....

SATURDAY ....

SUNDAY ....

MEAL PLAN FOR THE WEEK OF:

BREAKFAST IDEAS

LUNCH IDEAS

SHOPPING LIST

SO TASTY!

MONDAY . . . .

TUESDAY . . . .

WEDNESDAY . . . .

THURSDAY . . . .

FRIDAY . . . .

SATURDAY . . . .

SUNDAY . . . .

MEAL PLAN FOR THE WEEK OF:

BREAKFAST IDEAS

LUNCH IDEAS

SHOPPING LIST

BON APPÉTIT!

MONDAY ....

_____
_____
_____

TUESDAY ....

_____
_____
_____

WEDNESDAY ....

_____
_____
_____

THURSDAY ....

_____
_____
_____

FRIDAY ....

_____
_____
_____

SATURDAY ....

_____
_____
_____

SUNDAY ....

_____
_____
_____

MEAL PLAN FOR THE WEEK OF:

BREAKFAST IDEAS

LUNCH IDEAS

SHOPPING LIST

DELISH!

MONDAY
....

TUESDAY
....

WEDNESDAY
....

THURSDAY
....

FRIDAY
....

SATURDAY
....

SUNDAY
....

MEAL PLAN FOR THE WEEK OF:

BREAKFAST IDEAS

LUNCH IDEAS

SHOPPING LIST

NOM NOM NOM!

MONDAY ....

TUESDAY ....

WEDNESDAY ....

THURSDAY ....

FRIDAY ....

SATURDAY ....

SUNDAY ....

MEAL PLAN FOR THE WEEK OF:

BREAKFAST IDEAS

LUNCH IDEAS

SHOPPING LIST

SO TASTY! ▬▬▬

MONDAY . . . .

_____

_____

_____

TUESDAY . . . .

_____

_____

_____

WEDNESDAY . . . .

_____

_____

_____

THURSDAY . . . .

_____

_____

_____

FRIDAY . . . .

_____

_____

_____

SATURDAY . . . .

_____

_____

_____

SUNDAY . . . .

_____

_____

_____

MEAL PLAN FOR THE WEEK OF:

BREAKFAST IDEAS

LUNCH IDEAS

SHOPPING LIST

BON APPÉTIT!

MONDAY ....

_____

_____

_____

TUESDAY ....

_____

_____

_____

WEDNESDAY ....

_____

_____

_____

THURSDAY ....

_____

_____

_____

FRIDAY ....

_____

_____

_____

SATURDAY ....

_____

_____

_____

SUNDAY ....

_____

_____

_____

MEAL PLAN FOR THE WEEK OF:

BREAKFAST IDEAS

LUNCH IDEAS

SHOPPING LIST

DELISH!

MONDAY ....

TUESDAY ....

WEDNESDAY ....

THURSDAY ....

FRIDAY ....

SATURDAY ....

SUNDAY ....

MEAL PLAN FOR THE WEEK OF:

BREAKFAST IDEAS

LUNCH IDEAS

SHOPPING LIST

NOM NOM NOM!

MONDAY ....

TUESDAY ....

WEDNESDAY ....

THURSDAY ....

FRIDAY ....

SATURDAY ....

SUNDAY ....

MEAL PLAN FOR THE WEEK OF:

BREAKFAST IDEAS

_____
_____
_____
_____
_____
_____
_____
_____
_____

LUNCH IDEAS

_____
_____
_____
_____
_____
_____
_____
_____
_____

SHOPPING LIST

_____   _____
_____   _____
_____   _____
_____   _____
_____   _____
_____   _____
_____   _____
_____   _____
_____   _____
_____   _____
_____   _____
_____   _____
_____   _____
_____   _____
_____   _____
_____   _____

SO TASTY! ▬

MONDAY ....

_____
_____
_____

TUESDAY ....

_____
_____
_____

WEDNESDAY ....

_____
_____
_____

THURSDAY ....

_____
_____
_____

FRIDAY ....

_____
_____
_____

SATURDAY ....

_____
_____
_____

SUNDAY ....

_____
_____
_____

MEAL PLAN FOR THE WEEK OF:

BREAKFAST IDEAS

LUNCH IDEAS

SHOPPING LIST

BON APPÉTIT!

MONDAY
....

_____
_____
_____

TUESDAY
....

_____
_____
_____

WEDNESDAY
....

_____
_____
_____

THURSDAY
....

_____
_____
_____

FRIDAY
....

_____
_____
_____

SATURDAY
....

_____
_____
_____

SUNDAY
....

_____
_____
_____

MEAL PLAN FOR THE WEEK OF:

BREAKFAST IDEAS

_____
_____
_____
_____
_____
_____
_____
_____
_____

LUNCH IDEAS

_____
_____
_____
_____
_____
_____
_____
_____

SHOPPING LIST

_____	_____
_____	_____
_____	_____
_____	_____
_____	_____
_____	_____
_____	_____
_____	_____
_____	_____
_____	_____
_____	_____
_____	_____
_____	_____

DELISH!

MONDAY
....

TUESDAY
....

WEDNESDAY
....

THURSDAY
....

FRIDAY
....

SATURDAY
....

SUNDAY
....

MEAL PLAN FOR THE WEEK OF:

BREAKFAST IDEAS

LUNCH IDEAS

SHOPPING LIST

NOM NOM NOM!

MONDAY ....

TUESDAY ....

WEDNESDAY ....

THURSDAY ....

FRIDAY ....

SATURDAY ....

SUNDAY ....

MEAL PLAN FOR THE WEEK OF:

BREAKFAST IDEAS

LUNCH IDEAS

SHOPPING LIST

SO TASTY! ███████

MONDAY ....

_____
_____
_____

TUESDAY ....

_____
_____
_____

WEDNESDAY ....

_____
_____
_____

THURSDAY ....

_____
_____
_____

FRIDAY ....

_____
_____
_____

SATURDAY ....

_____
_____
_____

SUNDAY ....

_____
_____
_____

MEAL PLAN FOR THE WEEK OF:

BREAKFAST IDEAS

LUNCH IDEAS

SHOPPING LIST

BON APPÉTIT!

MONDAY ....

TUESDAY ....

WEDNESDAY ....

THURSDAY ....

FRIDAY ....

SATURDAY ....

SUNDAY ....

MEAL PLAN FOR THE WEEK OF:

BREAKFAST IDEAS

LUNCH IDEAS

SHOPPING LIST

DELISH! ▄▄▄▄▄▄▄

MONDAY . . . .

TUESDAY . . . .

WEDNESDAY . . . .

THURSDAY . . . .

FRIDAY . . . .

SATURDAY . . . .

SUNDAY . . . .

MEAL PLAN FOR THE WEEK OF:

BREAKFAST IDEAS

_____
_____
_____
_____
_____
_____
_____
_____

LUNCH IDEAS

_____
_____
_____
_____
_____
_____
_____
_____

SHOPPING LIST

_____   _____
_____   _____
_____   _____
_____   _____
_____   _____
_____   _____
_____   _____
_____   _____
_____   _____
_____   _____
_____   _____
_____   _____
_____   _____
_____   _____

NOM NOM NOM!

MONDAY ....

TUESDAY ....

WEDNESDAY ....

THURSDAY ....

FRIDAY ....

SATURDAY ....

SUNDAY ....

MEAL PLAN FOR THE WEEK OF:

BREAKFAST IDEAS

LUNCH IDEAS

SHOPPING LIST

SO TASTY! ■■■■

MONDAY . . . .

TUESDAY . . . .

WEDNESDAY . . . .

THURSDAY . . . .

FRIDAY . . . .

SATURDAY . . . .

SUNDAY . . . .

MEAL PLAN FOR THE WEEK OF:

BREAKFAST IDEAS

_____
_____
_____
_____
_____
_____
_____
_____
_____

LUNCH IDEAS

_____
_____
_____
_____
_____
_____
_____
_____
_____

SHOPPING LIST

_____   _____
_____   _____
_____   _____
_____   _____
_____   _____
_____   _____
_____   _____
_____   _____
_____   _____
_____   _____
_____   _____
_____   _____
_____   _____

BON APPÉTIT!

MONDAY ....

TUESDAY ....

WEDNESDAY ....

THURSDAY ....

FRIDAY ....

SATURDAY ....

SUNDAY ....

MEAL PLAN FOR THE WEEK OF:

BREAKFAST IDEAS

LUNCH IDEAS

SHOPPING LIST

DELISH!

MONDAY ....

TUESDAY ....

WEDNESDAY ....

THURSDAY ....

FRIDAY ....

SATURDAY ....

SUNDAY ....

MEAL PLAN FOR THE WEEK OF:

BREAKFAST IDEAS

LUNCH IDEAS

SHOPPING LIST

NOM NOM NOM!

MONDAY ....

TUESDAY ....

WEDNESDAY ....

THURSDAY ....

FRIDAY ....

SATURDAY ....

SUNDAY ....

MEAL PLAN FOR THE WEEK OF:

BREAKFAST IDEAS

_____
_____
_____
_____
_____
_____
_____
_____
_____
_____

LUNCH IDEAS

_____
_____
_____
_____
_____
_____
_____
_____
_____
_____

SHOPPING LIST

_____   _____
_____   _____
_____   _____
_____   _____
_____   _____
_____   _____
_____   _____
_____   _____
_____   _____
_____   _____
_____   _____
_____   _____
_____   _____
_____   _____
_____   _____
_____   _____
_____   _____

SO TASTY! ■■■■

MONDAY ....

_____

_____

_____

TUESDAY ....

_____

_____

_____

WEDNESDAY ....

_____

_____

_____

THURSDAY ....

_____

_____

_____

FRIDAY ....

_____

_____

_____

SATURDAY ....

_____

_____

_____

SUNDAY ....

_____

_____

_____

MEAL PLAN FOR THE WEEK OF:

BREAKFAST IDEAS

_____
_____
_____
_____
_____
_____
_____
_____
_____

LUNCH IDEAS

_____
_____
_____
_____
_____
_____
_____
_____
_____

SHOPPING LIST

_____   _____
_____   _____
_____   _____
_____   _____
_____   _____
_____   _____
_____   _____
_____   _____
_____   _____
_____   _____
_____   _____
_____   _____
_____   _____
_____   _____
_____   _____
_____   _____
_____   _____
_____   _____

BON APPÉTIT!

MONDAY ....

_____

_____

_____

TUESDAY ....

_____

_____

_____

WEDNESDAY ....

_____

_____

_____

THURSDAY ....

_____

_____

_____

FRIDAY ....

_____

_____

_____

SATURDAY ....

_____

_____

_____

SUNDAY ....

_____

_____

_____

MEAL PLAN FOR THE WEEK OF:

BREAKFAST IDEAS

LUNCH IDEAS

SHOPPING LIST

DELISH!

MONDAY ....

_____
_____
_____

TUESDAY ....

_____
_____
_____

WEDNESDAY ....

_____
_____
_____

THURSDAY ....

_____
_____
_____

FRIDAY ....

_____
_____
_____

SATURDAY ....

_____
_____
_____

SUNDAY ....

_____
_____
_____

MEAL PLAN FOR THE WEEK OF:

BREAKFAST IDEAS

LUNCH IDEAS

SHOPPING LIST

NOM NOM NOM!

MONDAY   . . . .

TUESDAY   . . . .

WEDNESDAY   . . . .

THURSDAY   . . . .

FRIDAY   . . . .

SATURDAY   . . . .

SUNDAY   . . . .

MEAL PLAN FOR THE WEEK OF:

BREAKFAST IDEAS

LUNCH IDEAS

SHOPPING LIST

SO TASTY! ▪▪▪▪▪▪

MONDAY ....

_____

_____

_____

TUESDAY ....

_____

_____

_____

WEDNESDAY ....

_____

_____

_____

THURSDAY ....

_____

_____

_____

FRIDAY ....

_____

_____

_____

SATURDAY ....

_____

_____

_____

SUNDAY ....

_____

_____

_____

MEAL PLAN FOR THE WEEK OF:

BREAKFAST IDEAS

LUNCH IDEAS

SHOPPING LIST

BON APPÉTIT!

MONDAY ....

_____
_____
_____

TUESDAY ....

_____
_____
_____

WEDNESDAY ....

_____
_____
_____

THURSDAY ....

_____
_____
_____

FRIDAY ....

_____
_____
_____

SATURDAY ....

_____
_____
_____

SUNDAY ....

_____
_____
_____

MEAL PLAN FOR THE WEEK OF:

BREAKFAST IDEAS

_____
_____
_____
_____
_____
_____
_____
_____

LUNCH IDEAS

_____
_____
_____
_____
_____
_____
_____
_____

SHOPPING LIST

_____ _____
_____ _____
_____ _____
_____ _____
_____ _____
_____ _____
_____ _____
_____ _____
_____ _____
_____ _____
_____ _____
_____ _____
_____ _____

DELISH!

MONDAY . . . .

TUESDAY . . . .

WEDNESDAY . . . .

THURSDAY . . . .

FRIDAY . . . .

SATURDAY . . . .

SUNDAY . . . .

MEAL PLAN FOR THE WEEK OF:

BREAKFAST IDEAS

LUNCH IDEAS

SHOPPING LIST

NOM NOM NOM!

MONDAY ....

_____

_____

_____

TUESDAY ....

_____

_____

_____

WEDNESDAY ....

_____

_____

_____

THURSDAY ....

_____

_____

_____

FRIDAY ....

_____

_____

_____

SATURDAY ....

_____

_____

_____

SUNDAY ....

_____

_____

_____

MEAL PLAN FOR THE WEEK OF:

BREAKFAST IDEAS

_____
_____
_____
_____
_____
_____
_____
_____

LUNCH IDEAS

_____
_____
_____
_____
_____
_____
_____
_____

SHOPPING LIST

_____   _____
_____   _____
_____   _____
_____   _____
_____   _____
_____   _____
_____   _____
_____   _____
_____   _____
_____   _____
_____   _____
_____   _____
_____   _____
_____   _____
_____   _____

SO TASTY! ██████

MONDAY
. . . .

TUESDAY
. . . .

WEDNESDAY
. . . .

THURSDAY
. . . .

FRIDAY
. . . .

SATURDAY
. . . .

SUNDAY
. . . .

MEAL PLAN FOR THE WEEK OF:

BREAKFAST IDEAS

LUNCH IDEAS

SHOPPING LIST

BON APPÉTIT!

MONDAY ....

_____

_____

_____

TUESDAY ....

_____

_____

_____

WEDNESDAY ....

_____

_____

_____

THURSDAY ....

_____

_____

_____

FRIDAY ....

_____

_____

_____

SATURDAY ....

_____

_____

_____

SUNDAY ....

_____

_____

_____

MEAL PLAN FOR THE WEEK OF:

BREAKFAST IDEAS

LUNCH IDEAS

SHOPPING LIST